The Broken Soldiers:
Suffering in Silence with Hidden Injury.

For security reasons, the names of the veterans in this book have been withheld.

"On the battlefield, the UK Armed Forces pledge to leave no soldier behind. As a nation, let it be our pledge that when they return home, we will look after our veterans."

The Contents

To all my family and friends who have supported me through a tough journey with my fight against Combat Stress aka PTSD. What follows wouldn't have happened if it wasn't for them.

Introduction

"Post-traumatic stress disorder (PTSD) is a mental disorder than can develop after a person is exposed to a traumatic event."

This is the Wikipedia description for PTSD. Anyone can look it up. Everyone knows that military personnel are likely to face difficult and challenging situations. You may think: 'Yes, I get that, God knows what these serving boys and girls have seen and been through.' You can try and imagine, but that is all you can do. I also did not understand, until I experienced first-hand the impact of PTSD.

Through the stories of six veterans, this book seeks to give insight into their broken hearts, bodies and minds – and the hell they experienced. This invisible hell of the traumatic sights, sounds, smells, screams, and pain cannot be forgotten and continues to haunt these veterans.

Nothing can make these experiences go away – that is impossible. But beyond their harrowing experiences, many veterans are let down by society even in this modern day. Their relationship with the world is forever changed. They return home to find they no longer fit into their former communities. Their loved ones may be unable to cope with or support these returning. The British government regularly turns its back on veterans suffering with Mental Health, reneges on its covenant, on its promises and on its duty to men and women who have lost so much through serving their duty.

Researching and writing this book has been an emotional rollercoaster. It is painful to see how our troops have been badly let down on so many levels not just by governments but also charities too. The pain, trauma and sense of betrayal are all tangible in the personal accounts of veterans battling PTSD. The subsequent disintegration of personal relationships is complex and at times happens around issues that cannot be controlled.

This book seeks to explain the challenges of PTSD to all who have not been there, who struggle to understand and seek to support those affected. We hope that this book has a wide and far reaching audience and inspires crucial changes that will make a positive difference in the lives of veterans and their loved ones.

"Even in times of trauma, we try to maintain a sense of normality until we no longer can. That, my friends, is called surviving. Not healing. We never become whole again ... we are survivors. If you are here today... you are a survivor. But those of us who have made it through hell and are still standing? We bear a different name: Warriors."

— Lori Goodwin

The Beginning

Throughout history in the UK, there has always been a terrible stigma hanging over mental health. Unfortunately, mental health continues to be a misunderstood topic. Doctors receive minimal training in this field and are often underprepared to effectively address mental health issues. Many people still have misconceptions regarding mental health, how and why it affects individuals and how to act. If we were to go back less than 100 years ago, anyone suffering from a mental health condition would have been locked up in a mental institution and most likely forgotten about, since this would have brought complete shame to their families. Treatment for mental health patients included horrific procedures such as lobotomies, trepanation, hydrotherapy and chemically induced seizures. Often these treatments left the patients like zombies and with permanent brain damage.

Today we have a greater understanding and openness to understanding and addressing a variety of mental health conditions. Post-Traumatic Stress Disorder (PTSD) is a form of mental illness that can develop after a person is exposed to one or more traumatic events throughout their life, such as sexual assault, warfare, road traffic accidents or any other form of traumatic events. In the case of veterans, this response is better known as 'Combat Stress.' Over the course of researching and writing this book and I conducted in-depth interviews with veterans who are suffering from combat stress.

Historically, there has been some awareness of the impact of combat stress. For example, William Shakespeare's' play *Henry V, Part 1,* written around 1597, includes a vivid and accurate description of the symptoms of PTSD. Yet we still struggle to accept and support people who are suffering from mental health in today's modern times. No matter what the conflict throughout history, there will always be casualties. Physical injuries are clearly obvious, but mental injuries can be more difficult to see and thus in some ways are more challenging to treat and support.

The public can understand physical injuries as they are visible for everyone to see, but those suffering from mental health injuries such as PTSD must live with the horrors of war forever with no cure.

''The Battles may be won by our brave troops of the UK Armed Forces in foreign fields, thousands of miles away from our green fields and peaceful countryside in the UK. But these brave troops are protecting our freedom, so we can live the wonderful life here in the UK far away from a hostile enemy''.

Operation Telic (Op TELIC)

Operation Telic (Op TELIC) was the codename for all the United Kingdom's military operations in Iraq, starting with the invasion on the 19th March 2003.

The eve of the war speech by the British Prime Minister Tony Blair on the *20th March 2003:*

"On Tuesday night, I gave the order for British forces to take part in military action in Iraq.

"Tonight, British servicemen and women are engaged from air, land, and sea. Their mission: to remove Saddam Hussein from power, and disarm Iraq of its weapons of mass destruction.

"I know this course of action has produced deep divisions of opinion in our country. But I also know the British people will now be united in sending our armed forces our thoughts and prayers. They are the finest in the world and their families, and all of Britain can have great pride in them.

"The threat to Britain today is not that of my father's generation. The war between the big powers is unlikely. Europe is at peace. The cold war already a memory.

"But this new world faces a new threat: of disorder and chaos born either of brutal states like Iraq, armed with weapons of mass destruction; or of extreme terrorist groups. Both hate our way of life, our freedom, our democracy

"My fear, deeply held, based in part on the intelligence that I see, is that these threats come together and deliver catastrophe to our country and world. These tyrannical states do not care for the sanctity of human life. The terrorists delight in destroying it.

"Some say if we act, we become a target. The truth is all nations are targets. Bali was never in the frontline of action against terrorism. America didn't attack al-Qaida. They attacked America.

"Britain has never been a nation to hide at the back. But even if we were, it wouldn't avail us.

"Should terrorists obtain these weapons now being manufactured and traded around the world, the carnage they could inflict to our economies, our security, to world peace, would be beyond our most vivid imagination.

"My judgment, as prime minister, is that this threat is real, growing and of an entirely different nature to any conventional threat to our security that Britain has faced before.

"For 12 years, the world tried to disarm Saddam; after his wars in which hundreds of thousands died. UN weapons inspectors say vast amounts of chemical and biological poisons, such as anthrax, VX nerve agent, and mustard gas remains unaccounted for in Iraq.

"So, our choice is clear: back down and leaves Saddam hugely strengthened; or proceed to disarm him by force. Retreat might give us a moment of respite but

years of repentance at our weakness would, I believe, follow.

"It is true Saddam is not the only threat. But it is true also - as we British know - that the best way to deal with future threats peacefully, is to deal with present threats with results.

"Removing Saddam will be a blessing to the Iraqi people. Four million Iraqis are in exile. Sixty per cent of the population is dependent on food aid. Thousands of children die every year from malnutrition and disease. Hundreds of thousands have been driven from their homes or murdered.

"I hope the Iraqi people hear this message. We are with you. Our enemy is not you, but your barbarous rulers.

"Our commitment to the post-Saddam humanitarian effort will be total. We shall help Iraq move towards democracy. And put the money from Iraqi oil in a UN trust fund so that it benefits Iraq and no one else.

"Neither should Iraq be our only concern. President Bush and I have committed ourselves to peace in the Middle East based on a secure state of Israel and a viable Palestinian state. We will strive to see it done.

"But these challenges and others that confront us - poverty, the environment, the ravages of disease - require a world of order and stability. Dictators like Saddam, terrorist groups like al-Qaida, threaten the very existence of such a world.

"That is why I have asked our troops to go into action tonight. As so often before, on the courage and determination of British men and women, serving our country, the fate of many nations' rests.

"Thank you."

Date: 19th March 2003

Time: 0630hrs (Local)

Location: Form Up Point (FUP) 'Barnsley' - Kuwait/Iraq Boarder

---

THIS WAS IT; MORE TO THE POINT IT WAS WAR. IT HAD STARTED AND WE WERE PUT ON 5 MINUTES NOTICE TO MOVE.

We had spent the past two months sitting around in the Kuwaiti desert, doing vehicle convoy drills, driving around for days, getting stuck in the sand and spending what seem like hours digging our vehicles free only to get stuck again only a few minutes later. This endless waiting felt soul destroying. It felt like a remake of the classic war film (1958) *'Ice Cold in Alex'* with Sir John Mills, only there was `NO COLD BEER` waiting for us at the end! If we weren't doing vehicle convoy drills, we were on the ranges shooting at wooden targets at 25 meters in the middle of the desert or sitting around waiting for orders or something to happen. I had already spent months like this in BATUS (*British Army Training Unit Suffield, Canada*) out on the prairies throughout my military career, and felt these endless drills were pointless.

Everyone wanted to get on with the job we came to do, but still no one knew if we were going into Iraq or even more to the point if Saddam would back down. It was without any doubt a waiting game, and a boring one at that.

That morning I had wakened to the cloudless blue sky of the Kuwaiti desert. The air felt fresh and the sun warmed on our faces. Finally, a day in the desert where it wasn't overcast, cold or raining. Everyone seemed to be happy and going about their daily morning routine. Vehicles, tents and personnel were spread out as far as the eye could see. The *BBC World Service* played from the vehicle radios. There was a smell of coffee in the morning air. Some of the people were cooking their breakfast; while others headed off to eat breakfast in one of the big white British Army catering tents with not a care in the world.

Suddenly shouts rang across camp: "Gas, gas!"
Vehicle horns were sounded to warn of an incoming attack. People banged metal on metal as a further warning. Everyone rushed to put on their issued *S10 Respirators* (gas masks) and take cover behind anything to protect them from the incoming Scud missile. We waited for the blast on impact. What the hell was happening? I was scared shitless with many different thoughts running around in my head. *Will I live to see my family and loved ones again? Will I live to see the day out?* We had no idea what was about to happen.

These Scud attack alerts were to be become part of everyday life throughout the start of the war. It seemed someone at Battle Group Headquarters (BGHQ) through it was funny to keep us on high alert - or perhaps they were just as bored as us and need a laugh from time to time.

- *20 Minutes until IMPACT... I guess the Iraqi Army just woke up and thought about sending us a Scud missile. How very nice of them...*

- *15 Minutes until IMPACT... Time for a quick brew and smoke before I die?*

- *10 Minutes until IMPACT... Hmmmm, I'm getting bored of waiting. Time for another cheeky smoke?...*

- *5 Minutes until IMPACT... I'm seriously getting bored HURRY UP; I have things to be doing!*

- *1 Minutes until IMPACT... All call signs stand down, false alarm. Really? You are joking at Battle Group Headquarters. Thanks,*

We simply sat there with our respirators on top of our heads, laughing and watching people run into a 12x12 army issue tent for protection. I wasn't sure what a tent would do under these circumstances, but it was still funny to watch. To me it seemed pointless to run for cover or put on our respirators if we were going to die. One thing was sure – we didn't know when anything was going to happens to us if it happened or well. We adapted the attitude of making the most of our time, and generally became a

Pain as they were nothing to but laugh and not taking anyone too seriously.

Finally, after sitting around for ages - orders came through from BGHQ. We were ordered to set off into Iraq. Now it was our time – our war was about to start. I cannot explain how I felt, but suddenly my military training took over. I felt an adrenaline rush like I'd never felt before in my life. I felt scared but very focused on the job at hand. Our convoy headed north towards the Iraqi border. We were moving up 'Route Tampa'. It was late afternoon. Off to our left, in the distance, I could see the burning oil fires in southern Iraq image that will stay with me forever. The air was thick with the smell of burning oil and the sound of jets and helicopters flying over top nonstop. As we came closer to the border of Iraq, the traffic became slower. It was a logistical nightmare with all the coalition forces heading north at once. It seemed everyone wanted a piece of the war and to be the first ones over the border into Iraq before it was all over.

Lucky me, I had been placed on top cover, standing with my head and torso above our truck canopy, ready to defend our vehicle with a rifle, not liking the odds if we were attacked. I was informed that my anticipated survival time as the top cover during the invasion was about two and half minutes once we crossed the border into Iraq.

The feeling I had while on top cover were the scariest moments of my life won't lie. I knew my life could be over in a matter of minutes once I crossed into Iraq. As we approached the first berm close to the border, our convoy drove past the old UN compound on the right. The compound had been deserted a couple of days prior to the invasion. I remembered watching the UN vehicles driving south past our camp a couple of days earlier as they returned into Kuwait City.

As we came closer to the border, the air became much thicker with black smoke from the burning oil fields. The smell was unlike anything I had smelled before in my life. This was it – we crossed the border though a huge berm with a gap dug out by the Royal Engineers. Suddenly all became real. This was its Iraq. Who knew what lay ahead, but it wasn't to be giggles, that was for sure?

.

Shellshock or PTSD?

The realities of war are often misrepresented in public opinion. One may hear people saying: ''I wasn't scared, it's my job'' or "It's what I had signed up to do.'' To be completely honest, that is complete rubbish. If you're not scared when going to war, there is something seriously wrong with you.

When you go into any war zone, it is a very strange experience because you must recognize that you are basically already dead. This is hardly a normal human feeling. No one tells you how to feel, but strangely enough everyone around you seems to feel this way too. It a very strange feeling, but I guess it is how we get the job done in the first place. This is most likely where the black humor of the military comes from... I can remember the night we crossed into Iraq from Kuwait. I could feel the adrenaline pumping through my body. I was scared and hyper alert, ready for anything to happen.

Around midnight, our convoy passed an Iraqi farmer just standing by the side of the road. He looked at us as if he didn't have a clue what was going on or why we were there. What does one do in these moments? Even with our differences, we are simply human. We gave him some food, water and continued onwards with our war to Basra.

Not until after it was all over, did I look back and reflect on these moments. It seemed like all this had never happened; it was such a distant memory in my head. It takes time for the body to register what we have experienced. For some, this may happen right away. For others it can takes days, months or even years to process certain experiences. Now years later, I still often wonder what happened to that Iraqi farmer.

Every war comes with the cost of human casualties. For some families their son, daughter, husband, wife or loved one may never return home as they have been killed in action doing a job they believed in and loved doing. Other veterans returning home from the battlefield may suffer visible physical injuries such as missing limbs or scars. Everyone can see these injuries and understandably will feel sorry for these veterans. However, other veterans returning home may not even look injured, yet may still be casualties of war. These casualties have a wound that is hidden within their minds.

The mental and emotional trauma of conflict continues in these casualties long after returning home from war. This hidden wound is called Post Traumatic Stress Disorder (PTSD) aka Combat Stress. PTSD comes with symptoms that are truly awful and those suffering will have these symptoms long after returning home if not for life. PTSD can be managed but cannot be cured.

Symptoms of PTSD:

- Work-related problems,
- Relationship problems,
- Feeling numb and empty,
- Feeling suicidal,
- Self-harm tendencies,
- Self-destructive tendencies,
- Being easily moved to tears,
- Avoidance of people,
- Avoidance of places,
- Panic attacks,
- Anxiety,
- Depression,
- Mood swings,
- Feeling isolated,
- Frequent periods of being withdrawal into oneself,
- Nightmares,
- Flashbacks,
- Insomnia,
- Night terrors, waking up covered in sweat,
- Anger or aggressive behavior,
- Feeling distrustful and suspicious,
- Blaming others,
- Misuse of alcohol, drugs, gambling and food,
- Seeking out high-risk dangerous pursuits.

Living with PTSD can have a shattering effect on people's lives. Medical understanding of PTSD is growing, but treatment and management remains challenging. Yet even with this progress, some people still have massive misconceptions and stigma regarding mental health. Why is the expression of mental health realities still seen as a sign of weakness?

Even the Ancient Greeks observed signs and symptoms of PTSD in their soldiers in 6th century BCE. PTSD is hardly a new injury from the battlefields; it has been with us humans since the day we started to be at war with each other. With new age technology and modern-day warfare, it would be nice to think PTSD will become an injury of the past. However, it appears that where wars being fought today there is still a need for boots on the ground. So, PTSD is an injury that will continue to be with us in the future and forever.

Conflict and violence remain part of our reality. The only year since the end of World War Two where no British Military Personnel were killed in a military conflict (KIA) was 1968 it would 51 years until this would happen again in 2016 and again in 2019. Since 1969 with the troubles in Northern Ireland (Operation Banner), approximately 2273+ British Military personnel have been killed in action (March 2016). In addition, there have been countless injured British Military personnel, but these figures are not publicly available. Tragically, there are many more veterans who suffer in silence from the hidden wound of PTSD. For a variety of reasons, many of these veterans haven't received help or support in managing the mental health challenges caused by their time in the military. Some of these veterans may not believe there is any support out there for them in civvy street. Some may simply think they are fine, unaware they are suffering from PTSD and struggling to live a normal life.

While researching and writing this book I came across some shocking and saddening stories while interviewing British veterans and their families. Other nations like the USA, Canada and Australia have taken steps to develop a veterans' welfare system that supports their veterans regardless of their injuries and guarantees lifetime support. Why has the UK not taken similar action to support their veterans? The USA and Australian learned a hard but important lesson after the Vietnam War, which came with a huge price regarding veterans' welfare. Today it seems the UK is having the same problem with veteran's welfare as the USA or Australia experienced after that Vietnam war. British troops have been involved in numerous major conflicts since 1945. Yet the help and support for these veterans is lacking. In the UK we have been conditioned to keep a stiff upper lip and to see mental health as a sign of weakness. This attitude has resulted in many veterans suffering in silence.

The Military Covenant was re-introduced in 2000, and it establishes mutual obligations between the nation and its Armed Forces even know it always been there since 1953. According to a national newspaper "it is an informal understanding, rather than a legally enforceable contract, but it is nevertheless treated with great seriousness within the services." In April 2000, the Military Covenant entered political discourse as a way of measuring whether the government and society have met their obligations to support members of the armed forces. The Military Covenant is a term used mainly by the British Military and the media in relation to the safeguards, rewards, and compensation for military personnel who risk their lives obeying military orders based on the policies of the elected civilian government. The Covenant argues that armed forces personnel should expect to be treated fairly by the Crown and expect the support of the nation and the government.

The Ministry of Defence has said: "In putting the needs of the Nation first, the British Military forgo some of the rights enjoyed by those outside the Armed Forces. So, at the very least, British Service Personnel should always expect the UK and their commanders to treat them fairly, to value and respect them as individuals and to sustain and reward them and their families." But throughout the UK many veterans are turned away from medical treatment or housing, contrary to the promises of the Military Covenant. Some council staff have never even heard of The Military Covenant, so they are hardly likely to support it.

The UK 'Soldering - Armed Forces Covenant' published in 2000 states:

"Soldiers will be called upon to make personal sacrifices – including the ultimate sacrifice –; in the service of the Nation. In putting the needs of the Nation

and the Army before their own, they forego some of the rights enjoyed by those outside the Armed Forces. In return, British soldiers must always be able to expect fair treatment, to be valued and respected as individuals, and that they (and their families) will be sustained and rewarded by commensurate terms and conditions of service. In the same way, the unique nature of military land operations means that the Army differs from all other institutions and must be sustained and provided for accordingly by the Nation. This mutual obligation forms the Military Covenant between the Nation, the Army, and each soldier; an unbreakable common bond of identity, loyalty, and responsibility which has sustained the Army throughout its history. It has perhaps its greatest manifestation in the annual commemoration of Armistice Day, when the Nation keeps covenant with those who have made the ultimate sacrifice, giving their lives in action".

In short, the UK Armed Forces Covenant expresses the moral obligation that the government and nation owe to the Armed Forces who sacrifice personal freedoms and often face dangerous situations. So, if a veteran is suffering or not coping after leaving the military what can he or she do? There are some remarkable military charities working with veterans and serving personnel of the British Military. Unfortunately, many veterans are not aware of what is available to them though these charities. While researching and writing this book, many of the partners and wives of the veterans that I interviewed commented on how difficult it is that they cannot ask for help on behalf of their loved ones. A number of these military charities state that the veteran must make the first contact, as this is seen as the first step in their road to recovery. But many military personnel and veterans won't ask for help as it goes against their pride. Left without support, some veterans are unable to reintegrate into civilian life and end up going through immense personal challenges, living on the streets or even in prison due to their PTSD and reliving the horrors of war.

There are very few veterans' welfare charities in the UK who specialize in mental health. They are underfunded and underprepared to cope with the numbers of veterans seeking help. For the 40 years, the British Military has been involved in every conflict around the globe. It was simply a matter of time before this mental health crisis happened. After all, military personnel are human, even if the military would prefer to regard individuals as numbers who can be replaced and forgotten. As one veteran commented: "Veterans' mental health is a ticking time bomb; the pin has been pulled and we are waiting for the explosion."

While researching and writing this book, I interviewed a veteran who was suffering from severe PTSD. I was shown around his small flat which had limited furniture and bare walls. In the kitchen I was shocked to discover he only had a couple tins of soup and a half-eaten loaf of bread in his food cupboard. When I asked him about the scarcity of food in his kitchen, he just looked at me and said: "I cannot remember the last time I had a homemade cooked meal.'' He then went on to tell me he had been waiting to hear if he would qualify for his war pension as he hadn't been able to work for many years due to suffering from PTSD. After we finished the interview, I shared what I knew about organisations that offer help and support to veterans like him. This veteran had to suffer alone for over ten years before learning about what supports are available to him. Paradoxically, he didn't hear this from the military or government he served for years, but from another veteran suffering from PTSD.

The term PTSD first appeared in 1980 in the third edition of the Diagnostic and Statistical Manual of Mental Disorders published by the American Psychiatric Association. The addition of this diagnosis is associated with the legacy of the Vietnam War disaster where numerous veterans returned home to insufficient support. Earlier conflicts had led to other names such as 'soldier's heart', 'shell shock' and 'war neurosis'. The term shell shock was first used during World War 1 and was first discussed in an article in 1915 by Charles Myers in the medical journal The Lancet.

The term shell shock was used widely by senior generals of the British Military during World War One to describe troops who showed signs or symptoms of what we now understand as PTSD. Due to the misconceptions of the medical and military establishment, soldiers exhibiting signs of PTSD were considered weak or cowardly. During World War One, some soldiers suffering from shell shock were put on trial for military crimes such as desertion and cowardice in the face of the enemy. Some of these trials resulted in the soldiers being executed by firing squad. A Royal Commission Report during World War One on shell shock stated it was a sign of weakness; therefore, it was not found in a good unit on the front line. The continued pressure to avoid medical recognition of shell shock meant that it was not considered a legitimate defense or diagnosis.

When the medical trains carrying battlefield casualties from the western front arrived back in the UK during World War One, soldiers suffering from shell shock were always in the last carriage. These carriages had been specially designed with no windows so that soldiers affected by shell shock were kept away from other casualties and did not infect them on the journey home. The unfortunate these soldiers suffering from shell shock would be offloaded last. Other soldiers received a hero's welcome home from the public, but the government believed it was in the public interest not to see these shell-shocked soldiers. The government feared this could damage morale and reduce public support for our brave troops fighting on the foreign fields. In short, it was not the British way to admit that our brave fighting soldiers weren't coping with stress and trauma of war.

By 1939 well over 120,000 veterans from World War One who had been awarded primary psychiatric disability were still drawing pensions – about 15% of all pensioned disabilities. Some were receiving pensions for 'soldier's heart' or 'effort syndrome', but the military did not proactively acknowledge the emotional and mental cost of war. At the beginning of World War Two, the term shell shock was banned by the War Office (MoD). The term *post concessional syndrome* was used to describe the traumatic response to the battlefields. This term was used by the British

Military until 1961, when *post concessional syndrome* was changed to *accident neurosis*. The real causes of the condition remained unclear and underexplored.

Until recently the British Military did not recognise the many soldiers, sailors and airmen who were suffering from what is known today as PTSD. These individuals have served in global conflicts ranging from Northern Ireland, the Falklands War, the First Gulf War, Bosnia, Kosovo, Afghanistan and Iraq. Upon their return, it was easy to dismiss the service personnel as being tired from combat and thus their mental injuries went undiagnosed. Whether these individuals carried on with their military careers or left the military, often their lives fell apart due to suffering from PTSD with inadequate or nonexistent support.

More recently, the British Military has taken some steps to mitigate PTSD after returning from an operational theatre of conflict. For the past 15 years or so, all British Military personnel returning home from overseas conflicts have participated in mandatory decompression. Personnel spend two days in debriefs, or in true squaddie style, drink plenty of beer which usually leads to fighting each other before heading back to the UK. This decompression time is seen as a way of letting off steam among military personnel and reducing the risk of PTSD and other forms of mental health injuries. While this two-day decompression period has some positive impacts, it is not an adequate preventative measure to PTSD and still leaves many military personnel sufferings in silence for fear of losing their military careers.

One difference between present day conflicts and historical conflicts such as both World Wars is that today a relatively small portion of the population is involved in the military. Many of the people who fought during these World Wars or did national service likely knew each other before enlisting in the military, potentially would demob together and would return to communities with others who had shared similar experiences. These veterans would go to work together, talk about their military experiences with comrades, and meet up in their local pub to enjoy a pint and good old smoke as a way of processing their experiences.

Sadly, most veterans today don't have the option of going into work and offloading to a work colleague in civvie street. Most likely their colleagues haven't been in the military and therefore do not understand what the veteran has been through. This leaves veterans isolated and without enough social support to process the trauma of war. Over time this can lead to veterans becoming seriously ill with mental health issues from PTSD. This leads to potentially massive consequences in their lives and often also impacts families with negative ripple effects. Does a two-day decompression break work for our troops returning home from modern day conflicts? Likely time will give us some answers, but in the meantime the British Government has not been ready for the flood of serving personnel and veterans coming forward suffering from PTSD or other forms of mental health challenges.

Worst Symptom - Suicide

On an Saturday evening in June 2015. I was home alone, and my mind was running wild. I was sitting in the living room watching a documentary about the war in Afghanistan. Suddenly it was like a 3D movie. I was there in the documentary – I could feel the heat and blast of the engines of the US Blackhawk Helicopters as they went past on the screen. I could taste and smell the sand. I was there again with the sweat and dust on my face. How could this be happening? These sensations overpowered me, I zoned out from the real world around me. Then suddenly I was back again in my living room. It all was becoming too overwhelming, and I couldn't cope. I had no idea what was happening to me.

The next part is what a friend informed me happened: That evening I had been texting my friend some truly dark thoughts. I felt cheated of my life and felt I should have died on the battlefield. My friend who I had been texting that evening drove over to my house because she was so worried, that I would do something terrible to myself. she decided to climb over my back gate and somehow managed to get into the kitchen. I had two dogs at the time, not guard dogs, more likely to welcome you with a smile and lick you to death.

Next thing I remember was waking up in the hospital thinking what I have done. Why was I here with drips and lines hanging out of me and with two police officers standing at the end of my bed? I looked over to see my friend sitting there looking worried as I wasn't going to wake but only to see her amazing smile. All I could do was cry, something I have not been able to do in years. I couldn't talk, I couldn't find the words to say sorry I could only just cry.

Suicide is by far the worst symptom of PTSD. I have witnessed the consequences first-hand, and I'm fully aware of what damage it can do to a person, and family and friends as well. Some people may say suicide is a very selfish act, but I totally disagreed. I never thought I would be someone who tried to take my life, not once but over half dozen attempts in the summer of 2015. I couldn't understand why I was attempting suicide. I'd had an amazing life. Not until I started Cognitive Behavioral Therapy (CBT) to manage my problems did I examine how PTSD was affecting my thinking and actions.

''Some studies suggest that suicide risk is higher among those who experienced trauma due to the symptoms of PTSD.''

www.ptsd.va.gov

Here was the answer I been seeking since I started writing this book:

"Frequent, vivid flashbacks and disruptions in day to day functioning may predispose people with PTSD to suicide. Severe anxiety-related symptoms such as irritability, jitteriness, and agitation may indicate a greater suicide risk."

www.everydayhealth.com

PTSD is a hidden injury that can sneak up on you. Before you know it, your life has forever changed for the worse. Regardless what you say to people or how you behave, they just think of you as someone who has become a complete nasty person, who hates everyone and life. Worst of all, you hate yourself. This battle cannot be won or cured, but I strive to manage my PTSD and help other people to understand.

Name of this book?

I wanted to give this book a name to remember, but I wasn't sure what to call it. So, I put this question out to the veterans whose stories are collected in this book. In late 2015 we were all talking via social media. We came up with countless names, some perhaps too offensive, and we finally decided on this title.

After reading the stories of these veterans one can only begin to understand the hardships they have faced and how determined they are to make a change in their lives. These stories also demonstrate how hard it is for individuals to carry on with the fight against PTSD. It can be a lonely journey against all odds, but regardless of the obstacles, these brave veterans have not given up. With each setback, the fight within them only grows stronger and stronger, even though they know there no cure for this injury. This courage is the sign of a true hero.

While researching and writing this book, I encountered veterans who I would consider the bravest people I have met in my life. I am proud to have served with them in the British Army and applaud their courage in coming forward to share their stories of PTSD. Fighting this battle, it is without any doubt the highest form of bravery. No one wants to admit they are suffering from mental health issues, and this is made even more difficult when the military and society are not supportive or understanding. As a nation we need to be more proactive in educating people about mental health. Simplistic films, sensationalistic media and antiquated social expectations in the UK continue to fuel misconceptions about mental health.

For those who are fighting combat stress, coming forward and asking for helping is true courage. For those suffering from this hidden injury, their battles will continue until the day they die. Some veterans suffering from PTSD will go on to live a semi-normal life, as they will be able manage and control their triggers. This will help them back into full- time work and family life. For many other veterans, their life won't be the same ever again. They remain unable to work and must live off a minimal war pension and inadequate state benefits. Even with this meagre support system, veterans with PTSD are determined to continue the fight no matter what. Some veterans are at peace with themselves, are thankful for what little support they receive, and will continue to live life not knowing any better. Some veterans will never talk about what trauma they have witnessed in combat and will not even admit to having served in the military. Some veterans have lost faith in the military and feel betrayed by their country. It is only a matter of time before too many of these veterans isolate themselves and are no longer able to participate in the community. Every bang or startling noise sends them back to the war zone, potentially causing them to do something dangerous to themselves or others. The standard of care for veterans' welfare is not much better than it was after World War One. Now 100 years later, why do we still expect veterans to recover from mental and emotional trauma with little or no help?

From a personal perspective, I don't care who knows that I have PTSD. I am open about how it has impacted my life. I have learned not to hide behind the injury as ignoring the need for treatment causes more damage than good. Some people may think of me differently, and some people may not understand regardless how long I have known them! Again, these reactions go back to the stigma around mental health. Some people are scared to understand mental health and think you should be locked up for life out of the public view. The friends that do stand by you through these ups and downs are the ones who care. Some of them may not understand but are still be there for you, and these are true friends. Such true friends are very rare. Regardless of what people think about veterans with PTSD, we are still the same people, no matter what happens in life or on the battlefield. As a nation, we need to support the veterans who have put their lives on the line for us to live a life of freedom.

The Broken Soldiers:
Suffering in Silence with Hidden Injury.

"Let US help you to understand Post Traumatic Stress Disorder Aka Combat Stress, and hopefully you will help us to fight and support the ones who are suffering. This is all we ask"... Soldier No.4

The following are the true personal accounts of six veterans of the UK Armed Forces, all of whom are suffering from PTSD. These six veterans have served with the UK Armed Forces in some of the world's worst modern-day conflicts since the end of World War two.

These accounts are true and have been written by the veteran themselves. Putting their experiences into words is a form of treatment in their road to recovery and enables others to understand how they feel and what they have witnessed during their military careers. It has been hard for these veterans to revisit their experiences, but they have done it in the hope it will help others to understand. Most importantly, these personal accounts are intended to show other veterans that you are not alone, and help is out there.

Military personnel must adopt a 'NOT CARING ATTITUDE' throughout their military career, especially while one is on operation tour. Without this 'NOT CARING ATTITUDE' personnel would not be able to do their job, but this leaves no space for processing experiences and trauma. Soldiers experience a lot more trauma than most, and over much longer periods of time. Ultimately this has consequences for their mental and emotional wellbeing. This is costs are demonstrated by chilling facts; for example, more veterans have killed themselves since returning home from the Falklands War in 1982 than the 255 that were killed in action.

All military personnel must adopt a 'NOT CARING ATTITUDE' at some point throughout their military career. If they didn't, they wouldn't be able to do their job in the first place. If they went around thinking they're going to die no one would join the Armed Forces. 'NOT CARING ATTITUDE' has always been the best policy in the context of the military. However, with this attitude, military personnel do not have an easy time of it in civvie street after leaving the military. Some veterans reintegrate into civilian life somewhat easily while others can't cope without the support network they once have in the military. Some veterans think their pride, career or reputation will be at risk if they ask for help.

Military personnel today see more combat and have more opportunity to kill the enemy than their grandfathers did in the Second World War or Korea. Then there was an army of over a million, spread over several continents during post-war Britain. Now military personnel experience combats almost every day while on operational tour. Military personnel affected by PTSD are casualties of war just as much as soldiers who lose limbs, are shot or hit by an I.E.D. Insufficient recognition of this mental health crisis is a ticking time bomb waiting to explode.

We as a nation must act now before it is too late to help those in need. We need a paradigm shift, where seeking help should be a sign of strength and professionalism, representative of the desire to maintain peak efficiency and wellbeing. The US Military have been doing this for years, and this is one factor that contributes to their powerful military force. War causes mental and emotional as well as physical wounds. We shouldn't be surprised by what can happen to military personnel who have seen combat. After all, they are human beings with feelings, hearts and minds. All military personnel and veterans need support, not just from the government but from society. There are underfunded charities that do their best to help veterans recover, but it's up to us to help remove the stigma around mental health. A little understanding can go a long way in supporting individuals battling difficult circumstances.

The following accounts may be upsetting to the reader, but they are the true accounts of veterans who are suffering from PTSD. Long after this book has been finished, these veterans will continue to be affected by PTSD until the day they die. These are the stories of their fight against PTSD.

Soldier - No. 1

"PTSD affects every person from the sufferer to the spouses to children to extended family."

It was through my own road to recovery that I came across a lot of people who don't understand mental health. As soon I mentioned I had PTSD, I could see that some people didn't understand. Some people became very judgmental and treated me like an alien from another planet. I'd been out of the army for a while, thinking I was living a semi-normal life. To be honest, I will never live a normal life on civvie street after leaving the army. Maybe it's because I'm just too regimental in many ways, or it's due to the black sense of humor that comes from being in military. I didn't know, and I didn't care. This attitude was to come back and bite me.

I hadn't been right well for a while, but my 'army head' was telling me that I was OK. I was waking up during the early hours of the morning with night sweats, having anger outbursts at home and at work, and drinking alcohol get to get blind drunk. These were textbook symptoms of PTSD. But I didn't want to admit to anyone that I had become 'weak'. After all, I was a veteran of Kosovo, Iraq and Afghanistan. People saw me as a role model and looked up to me. I didn't understand what was happening to me, even though I had seen and witnessed things that would give most people nightmares.

Why was it me that had to become ill with PTSD?

I blamed everyone around me for everything that was happening to me. In other words: *"I HATE CIVVIES"*. Only later did I learn how wrong I was about that attitude.

My story starts in 2003 with OP TELIC in Kuwait and Iraq. This was my first deployment to a war zone. Up until this point I had been living an amazing life in the army, with postings to Canada, Germany and Gibraltar. Something changed in me during my first deployment, though I wasn't aware of this change at the time. As the years passed, I became someone I wasn't. A lot of people started to hate me, but I didn't care. If anything, I would put 100% effort into my military career but not into my home life. This was my way of staying focused and trying to forget about what happen in Iraq. But this came with a huge price. The symptoms of PTSD from which I was suffering were becoming stronger. The stronger the symptoms became, the weaker I grew inside, and eventually PTSD took over who I was as a person.

In 2006, I was deployed out to Kosovo with my new unit. I was in a new job that put me under a lot of pressure. I became so focused on deploying out to Kosovo that my married life fell apart. Yet I didn't give a care about that or anyone else for that matter, apart from my military career.

I returned home from Kosovo a very hollow man, sad inside after witnessing how cruelly humans can treat each other in the 21st century. I felt numb and empty as a human. Within months of returning home, I had left my wife. One Sunday evening in early January 2007, I went out for a drink and never returned home, I didn't feel anything towards my ex-wife or anyone else in my life. As always, I just continued to soldier on. As the years passed. From the outside, my life looked amazing, but something was still missing. There was no adrenaline in my life aside from beating the rush hour traffic to and from work. I felt OK, but life seemed boring. PTSD took control of my life and I was drinking heavily. I didn't give a shit about home life. I was a squaddie, living the dream of being a soldier. But I missed the lifestyle of being on tour; part of me just wouldn't let it go. After all, this was my identity – why should I let it go?

In late 2011, I decided it was time to go back on tour, Afghanistan. I volunteered and told my partner and family I had been asked to deploy. *Excellent,* I thought, *I'm back where I belong – on tour.* I kept trying to explain to my ex-girlfriend that I needed the adrenaline rush in my life. This caused some long and heated arguments between us, but as always, I wouldn't listen. I was getting bored of being at home in fact I hated home life. I loved my family, but I felt that a regular nine to five job wasn't for me. In the combat zone I felt like the me agin, doing what I knew best and loved. For better words, I was home –

HOME SWEET HOME

March 2015, I had been out of the army 2 years and I hadn't noticed any changes in me, but everyone else had noticed it. Inside of me I had a ticking time bomb waiting to go BOOM. It was just a question of how long before it went off and what sort of damage and impact it would bring to me and everyone around me. It became a waiting game with the demons of PTSD.

My Formula for PTSD;

Kosovo + Iraq + Afghanistan + Drinking Heavily + Insomnia + Night Sweats + Night Terrors + Mood Swings + Arguing + Flashbacks + Suicidal Thoughts

= PTSD / COMBAT STRESS TIME BOMB

In the early summer of 2015, medical professionals informed me that if I didn't get help ASAP, I wouldn't live to see my 40th Birthday (2020) as there was a high chance of me taking my own life. The horrors of war haunted me daily, and I was suffering from flashbacks, night sweats, and suicidal thoughts. This was to become my own war, my war against the PTSD. Time was slipping away – I needed to move fast and get help before it was too late.

I felt like I was living life as *Jekyll and Hyde* – I never knew what to expect each morning when I woke up. If I had an argument with someone, I was not in control I felt like I was watching from the outside, unable to control myself – a very strange out of body experience. Not until after the arguments had finished would I start to get some control of the myself, but at that point it was too late. I would be left wondering what had just happened, with little memory of the argument and trying to piece together the puzzle. I felt like I became public enemy No.1 in the eyes of everyone around me. When I joined the army, the first thing we were taught in basic training was to attack every situation and never to retreat. Everyone has this fight or flight mode from the day we are born, however, the military trains their soldiers to fight and never flee, as this is how wars are won. This training doesn't help if you are suffering from PTSD during an argument – you will fight until you have won the argument, not understanding the value of different perspectives or perhaps walking away to let things calm down. It was also during these arguments the body produces the same adrenaline as being in battle, but there is no outlet for this adrenaline no pressure release. This causes PTSD to go into overdrive, and not until the adrenaline has dissipated does one become aware of surroundings and what has happened.

In the early summer of 2015, I went through the worst time of my life suffering from a PTSD breakdown. I lost my home. My relationship ended. I couldn't control my PTSD. I felt that my PTSD was winning the battle every step. On multiple occasions, I took countless overdoses as I didn't want to continue the fight anymore. I was tired of fighting this battle and wanted to be free. Many people around me saw these overdoses as a very selfish act but it wasn't to be, I was taking the overdoses to be at peace with myself and against the battle known as PTSD. I kept repeating the same question to myself time and time again.

Why me? What had I done wrong in my life to be suffering from PTSD?

Because of my actions from PTSD, I ended up sleeping on an air bed in my parents' living room and living out of a suitcase. Over time, I have learned to manage my battle and understand what is happening within me. I'm aware there no cure for PTSD, but more importantly I have again found the person I was before deploying to Iraq. I can once again start to enjoy life and there is light at the end of the tunnel. The train of PTSD has passed for the moment. It may return one day, but I will be ready to fight it head on. I have met many other veterans who are suffering from PTSD, not just from the UK but from around the world. We have formed a bond of friendship that is so stronger than the friends we made in the military.

,

NOTE: In the summer of 2015, I participated in sporting event at a military recovery center in Catterick. It was while staying at this center I shared a room with another veteran who had suffered a terrible injury in Afghanistan. He had been shot in the head. I couldn't even start to understand what he had to go through every day. One evening we were chatting, and I happen to mention too him: "I can't even image what you have been though or how you live every day with your injury." His reply was shocking and will live with me until the day I die. He turned, looked into my eyes and said: "I can see my injuries every day when I look in the mirror. I think to myself I'm lucky. But for you, you live a life with the hidden wound that you can't see when you look in the mirror. I wouldn't be able to live or cope with that. It must be the hardest thing to do – live life knowing you are carrying an injury which can't be seen or cured."

Soldier - No.2

I am now a victim of that despicable lie.

I was sitting in the MO office at the PRC. It was a run of the mill check-up. I had been ill with the flu for some time and I was feeling lousy. I had known the MO for over fifteen years. Our paths had crossed many times during my service in the army. After my check-up, the MO started to fill out my prescription. He paused and looked at me for a moment but didn't say anything. He did exactly like in the famous scene in the film *Good Will Hunting*. Except instead of saying: "it's not your fault," he repeated: "is there anything else?" By the fourth time he said it I had my nervous breakdown.

Over the years he had seen me at my best and worst and knew me quite well. Four hours later after seeing the Community Psychiatric Nurse and Psychiatrist, I was told to walk out of the building straight to my car and drive to my parents' house in the countryside. The MO had rung my parents and given them strict instructions to call him on my arrival to make sure I got home safely.

My journey had begun. For the last year, I have been on what is called recovery duty. I am not fit or well enough to go back to work. The last year has been the biggest battle of my military career. It has been uncharted waters.

It began nearly two decades ago in a place called Deepcut Barracks, Surrey, doing basic training in

Princess Royal Barracks. As a young soldier I knew no better and thought that was the army way.

I loved the first unit I was posted to and found it totally amazing. It was a big unit and like a family to me and everyone else in the unit. I soon found myself in Bosnia, and went to places like Goradze, Sipovo, Gorni Vakuf, and Mostar. We had our hands tied from taking action as we were with the UN and we came under very restricted rules of engagement. I witnessed things that no humans should see in their lifetime. It was disgusting to see what people did to each other in this conflict. Many years later, what I saw still haunts me to this day. It also feels like we were part of a forgotten conflict since we don't hear much about Bosnia anymore. Once the tour had the finished, we went straight home where we returned to the barracks and had no decompression.

I went back again to Bosnia two years later as part of NATO. This time we had less restricted rules and could fire back if we felt our lives were in danger. I was with a medical unit, so I saw a lot of severe injuries, accidents and murder victims. Again, I came back from tour with no decompression, debrief or mental health follow-ups.

While in Bosnia, I had on several occasions crawled through and cleared minefields to reach injured people and save them. It took me a long time to walk on the grass again after my second tour as it made me feel like I was walking on a mine field. Some of my work involved EOD disposal. Sometimes I was at arm's distance from a live mine or grenade, and in one instance a Hellfire missile.

I did three tours in Iraq. The first two were back to back. We were ambushed so often that I lost count. My crew was targeted by an IED team, and we were lucky not to be caught. However, another crew lost their lives to the same IED team and I lost several friends. In every operational theater I have ended up in the thick of the action. I am not an infantryman, just an REMF (Rear Echelon Motherfucker). But I must be a bullet magnet because I have probably seen and been part of more contacts than most infantrymen see in their career.

Things started to unravel several years ago when I was injured in a stupid accident. The army is designed to work with fit individuals. I had heard of PTSD but did not realize what it was. After a year, I am still learning about it and what it is doing to me. It's not a mental condition as lots of people think it is. It is a physical condition where your brain has endured too much traumatic stress and it rewires itself. Imagine you are about to do a bungee jump: your body fires out a ton of adrenaline, floods your body, you get giddy, your senses heighten, and your hearing, touch, smell and vision become superhuman. When you jump, that chemical kicks in and you get a high. Unfortunately, with PTSD that happens all the time, and it does not ever switch off. What did that do to me? I cannot leave the house to go to the shops. I instantly go into patrol mode; while a civilian can walk three yards and not think anything of it. For me, I'm looking for IEDs, vulnerable points, critical points, snipers, unusual sounds, movement. In those three yards, I am that soldier again.

Because of my PTSD, I get flashbacks, which are evil. It's like suddenly being transported back to Afghanistan and you react as if you're in Afghanistan. This does not stop when you go to sleep. Once I was woken by the sanitation workers outside, and instantly I was on the bedroom floor looking for my rifle. The smells of diesel, grass, copper and fecal matter give me flashbacks. My muscles are contracted all the time, and I am in constant pain; I fall over a lot and have become extremely clumsy. My social life has disappeared, and normal things have become more difficult. A trip to the shops may take three or four days. I have to steel myself to go out the front door. Outside of the routine that I have adopted, I become difficult when there is any change. My family has suffered; the normal bubbly person that I once was has gone. All they see is me and my cold stare and angry outbursts.

I have been placed on several courses run by the Royal British Legion and Help for Heroes. You must do them as part of your recovery journey. Some of it helps, but the overriding outcome is that you end up with people like yourself, and a support network grows out of that. While doing these courses, I was spotted by an Olympic coach from Team GB in a particular sport. I am now training for that sport, as a goal to achieve before leaving the army. My recovery center has given me some support, but I find charities like RBL and H4H are better at it. Help for Heroes has rescued me from myself. It hasn't cured me, but it's getting me to the point where I can leave in a better position. It's helping me with my career, sport and physical and mental well-being.

Recently I was at Tedworth House, the Help for Heroes recovery centre, sitting one evening at a table with other soldiers of varying rank, age, and experience. For that one night, I smiled, laughed and joked and felt safe. They immediately understood that I could not sit with my back to the window or the door. They knew when I was having a flashback and also how to bring me back. One thing a soldier has is banter, and for that one night, I was my old self. Help for Heroes has helped me leave the house, understand when I arrive, I am exhausted, and put me with the best people in the country.

If someone could make a panacea for PTSD, I would take it in a heartbeat. I sat with a triple amputee and felt bad that I was able bodied. When I told him so, with his false arm he put his hand on my knee and told me that he felt sorry for me. People can see his injuries and adjust, but people can't see PTSD, they cannot see the brain damage that you have. We totted up all the traumatic incidents that have affected me; it came close to twelve separate incidents, all of which were extremely disgusting and terrifying. As a soldier, we are trained to fight the repulsion and emotions that happen during these incidents. But later the body and mind will relive that moment over and over.

Well, it's been over a year since I wrote my chapter for this book, so here is an update. Being a soldier on the transition to Civvy Street is a daunting experience. As a soldier with multiple injuries and a mental health condition it's even worse.

The process was not easy. I had help from the Personnel Recovery Unit, who did what they could to help. But the second you walk out of the camp gates you are your own entity. Nothing can prepare you for that.

A further blow was that at the point of leaving, a private hospital discovered two injuries that I had sustained on military operations. One is life changing, the other is life threatening. The life-threatening injury was missed due to the low standard of medical care that I received while serving. The suck it up and fight attitude left me in the position that if lucky I will be a paraplegic for the rest of my life, or if unlucky, I will drown in my bodily fluid while paralyzed from the neck down.

The army covenant does not exist in Civvy Street. If you mention it, you are treated like you have two heads. Dealing with civilians is a nightmare. Punctuality is a big part of my PTSD, and they are always late, or if late fail to call. You have to chase people up all the time; you cannot trust anyone. Dealing with the War Pension takes a minimum of eight months to be sorted, leaving me massively out of pocket. I had to fight for Personal Independence Payment, which I should not have to had to do, but it has no provision for mental health conditions. I have yet to secure employment, which I know will be a fruitless exercise. Getting a job while disabled is a nightmare; keeping the same job with my mood swings is another story.

With the help of the guys who have written this book I feel a bit better and I understand myself more, but I still have wobbly moments. This morning the postman startled me. Three hours later I am still sitting on the sofa shaking. The symptoms are still there. I wait for my partner to leave in the morning, so I can take the bedding down to wash after my night sweats. The sudden flashbacks to Iraq or Bosnia still go on. I was cooking bacon the other day, and burnt it, and then without realizing it I was wandering around the living room looking for a burnt body. Some days I will be fine, and then suddenly I look at the front door and think I could just put my coat on and walk out. Other days I think about killing myself, I know I won't do it, but thinking about it calms me. I have walked out of shops leaving shopping in the basket, lost my temper while driving and drifted off when people are talking to me.

The other scary thing is when I try talking to anyone who is not ex-military, they don't understand that what I may have done in six months is more than they have done in six years. It's hard work. The upside is I am waiting for my stint at Combat Stress; it is a goal and something I need to do for my family and me. The Ministry of Defense has no aftercare or takes no responsibility for military personnel. It's akin to hiring a brand-new car and bringing it back dented and broken. If this happened, the hire firm would expect the damage to be paid for and sorted. I am the hire car that the MoD took responsibility for and they have now put me back on the market dented and broken. They just shrugged their shoulders and walked off without paying.

Soldier - No.3

Struggle back on Civvy Street with the fight against Combat Stress.

After tours in Kosovo, Iraq, and Afghanistan, I returned to my hometown of Ashington only to be diagnosed with Post Traumatic Stress Disorder (PTSD). Here, in my words, I will reveal my heart-breaking struggle to return to a normal life beyond the warzone.

There are twenty-six letters in our alphabet. Some of them can be strung together to denote disease, conditions, or just about any acronym we see fit to label people with. So, when I was given four of them, I wasn't surprised really. Although the way they were handed over was a bit of a kick in the teeth.

Growing up on the streets of Ashington in the 80s didn't exactly reward itself with too much merit. As soon as I could, I fled the Northeast to see if it was any better in other places around this great country of ours. There are no streets paved with gold, and I found we all have to make our own way through life eventually. At the tender age of 27, I left the comfort of civilian life and embarked on my wanderings around the world, wearing green and carrying a gun. I was a little older than the average recruit; in fact, I was the oldest there at that time. The fitness worried me a tad, being up against the teenagers who had been working hard to gain access to the military.

Basic training seemed to be entirely in the mindset of the individual - although we were under the illusion that the Army wasn't looking for individuals. Sailing through the 12-week chaff sorting, I came out the other end with a clear idea of what was expected of me.

Fifteen years, three stripes and three warzones later, I shrugged off the shackles of camouflage and dusted off the jeans and loud shirts. However, those 15 years left their scars. It wasn't until the end that they made their presence known to me - they had made themselves visible to everyone else much earlier.

My daughter was the first one to suffer the piercing blade of my wrath through an innocuous statement about training shoes. I screamed in her direction that there were people around the world who would love to wear shoes, but they couldn't as they had their legs blown away by Improvised Explosive Devices (IED's). My mood was black as my outlook on life now. It was due to Kosovo first, then Iraq, then finally Afghanistan, all in the space of six years. Normally soldiers have a training year, then a deployment year, then a stand down year, so an extra deployment wasn't considered any big deal within the structure.

The hidden cost of modern warfare are the soldiers that don't show scars, the guys and girls who come home with all limbs intact, with no holes in them, with no outward signs of injury. But unfortunately, what they have seen, experienced and dealt with is etched into their brains just as any physical scars of an enemy action.

When you look at a young military person with a physical disability, you might feel a bit proud that they have sacrificed something for their country. When you hear about a soldier that has beaten up his spouse or ended up in jail because of a drunken night, you think: 'he deserves it, the bastard', but you don't see what is in his - or her - head.

Inside my head is a blank, a missing part of my life that has been erased at the source to save me from the terror of what happened throughout my deployments.

2012 was my final year in green; the transition back to civilian life took and is still taking its time. Job after the job has come and gone with testing and re-adjusting at every angle. I first asked the system to help me gain employment in the education environment, but because I had spent my time as a mechanical engineer in the Royal Electrical and Mechanical Engineers (REME) I was told that teaching wasn't an option.

I was going to have to forge own my path to reach my goals... again. The tenets instilled during my employment by the Army held fast into civilian life - tenets such as respect, integrity, and loyalty to name but a few. Unfortunately, these seemed to be lacking in my chosen career outside the Army, ANY chosen career. Fitting in was going to be difficult it seemed, but I was determined to bring a sense of camaraderie to whichever path I decided to walk.

My anger slowly bubbled under the surface as new "triggers" were found, triggers of which I wasn't aware.

The whole point of my time under the Department of Community and Mental Health (DCMH) while still in the Army was to sort me out. It hadn't. I wasn't aware of still needing help. So, the fact I had no time for anyone didn't raise any red flags to me or anyone else in control.

I moved back to the Northeast to be near my family, then decided that a life abroad was the answer. Cyprus was a place I could be myself, a place where no one knew me personally, so I could be who I wanted to be. I could deviate from anything I was pigeon-holed for. I cleaned pools; I built fences, I painted houses, I became a diver. A whole new outlook took hold of me, and I thought I had left that another guy behind. At the end of the season I came back to the UK for the winter knowing I had a chance of a job the next season back in Cyprus. A few months later, I flew back to Cyprus. The guys in charge had changed and the clamoring urge to self-destruct raised its head again. Severing ties with the island, I flew to Sinai for another bite at the apple. I didn't want to come back to the UK at that time, so I continued my diving and made a life out there.

By 2012/13, I had decided that the red button in my life had to be pressed again, so I made my way to Hungary and a relationship that was built on eye contact under the waves of the Red Sea. My mind wanted to start something new, something different, another blank slate upon which to scribble another chapter of my life, but this time another person had noticed the cracks.

It was with heavy heart I had to admit defeat. My life was disappearing up its arse. If I kept on this course, who knows what would have happened? There are many stories of young people who are ex-military, ending up either banged up or worse. I rang the number I had for the UK arm of Combat Stress and appointments were made with outreach officers to see me at my temporary address (I was sleeping on my sister's couch).

Six weeks of intensive therapy in Scotland were prescribed - after the NHS decided that it could offer me nothing apart from a visit to the local mental institution - and I was released upon the civilized world again. My drive back to Ashington was interrupted by a plea to stop the car, so I could get out and howl my frustrations and trepidations at a fence along the A69.

Where I am now, compared to where I was before, has been only possible with help from new friends and people in the same situation. Trying to settle into a new flat with all the trappings of a "normal" life is still an ongoing process. Having to deal with trivial situations such as rubbish disposal, workers wanting to fix things that have nothing to do with you, noisy neighbors – in fact, everything that we aren't taught how to deal with in the Forces must be self-taught. If I had a problem with my room, I would ring the Quartermaster and ask them to sort it out. We're not taught how to deal with everyday life outside the security of the wire fence. We are taken from a civilian background and fettled into something resembling a soldier. We are taken to the height of our tolerance and taught to react in an aggressive manner to all situations.

We are constantly at the limit of our 'Red Button.' What isn't done is allowing us to come down from that height. We aren't told or taught how to climb down from that constant state of readiness. So, in any confrontational situation we find ourselves in, we react with the same red mist as we would respond to an enemy.

PTSD brings with it a watered-down reaction to ANYTHING that could even slightly resemble a trigger situation. I have had several encounters where, through no fault of their own, I have come close to throwing folk through plate glass windows because they transgressed some imagined line in my sand.

I don't look for trouble, I don't look for excuses, I signed on the dotted line to fight for Queen and Country, and I signed my life away for £15. I signed for what I thought was a 22-year enlistment with a pension and a lot of happy memories.

What I got was a bit different. I was not expecting to be living a life of horror behind the façade of a smile. I hide the fact that I want to scream and shout and lash out at every opportunity where I perceive danger lurking.

Throughout my time back in civilian life, I have kept an online diary, a diary I where can get what I am feeling out into the open. It's a cathartic pastime where I can see the ups and downs of my life in denim. I originally started it for my daughter Skye, so she can see that her dad is alive and well, but it has become a sounding board for my inner emotions, the feelings of rage and anger that aren't allowed in civilized life. Life is taken for granted by your average everyday guy or girl who wake up at a civilized time, get ready to do a day's work, enjoy some entertainment in the evening, and then go to bed.

Ask anyone who has seen things they shouldn't have. Ask anyone who has gone through hell and thought they were going to be fine with it all, how they start their day.

The big things don't matter - I've just lost my dad to stomach cancer - it's the little things that set my flame to incandescent. Someone not helping me when I know it's in their power, someone stopping me through ignorance from doing what I set out to do, something not quite going to plan when I have instinctively prepared everything.

Life is intrinsically hard anyway, but the mess left inside a soldier's head makes it virtually impossible. To some it IS impossible with only one outcome. I have had those thoughts, and it has taken me several attempts to dispel those, but the struggle is ongoing.

I have many people to thank for where I am today, not all on the positive, but with their help, I have only found myself. I will strive to achieve all I am able, and as I find other avenues, I will inform others in my position about what is available for them.

Life is complicated enough as it is – why make it harder by releasing soldiers without the tools needed for peace, but with ALL the tools for war still raging in their heads.

Soldier - No.4

Whoever fights monsters should see to it that in the process he does not become a monster. And if you gaze long enough into an abyss, the abyss will gaze back into you.

Friedrich Nietzsche

When a friend asked me to contribute to this book, I first felt didn't feel I had anything worthy to add.

This is not a war story at all but the real-life story of the cost of war. I do not want admiration, respect or sympathy. I am by no means a hero or a role model, but I am the waste product of what happens when humanity fails to see the futility of conflict.

I left the army in 2000, after being medically discharged due to damage to my legs. As far as service life goes, that's where this story ends. Yes, I have done tours and yes, I have looked into the abyss. I have done things I regret, and which are ever present in my waking hours and haunt me when I try to sleep.

Upon becoming a civilian, my transition was smooth. I got a job in the telecommunications industry and found myself working with former colleagues from my unit. Excellent, what else could I ask for? I was living not far from the base that I had once called home. The base was on the south coast of England, just a few miles from Portsmouth.

It was a great time. I lived with a girlfriend in a flat we had bought in the local area. Many of the lads who had left the Army had also settled in the area, so I had a good support network and was never alone when I needed to talk to someone. The years rolled on, as they do, and I moved to the southwest of England with a new job and a new start. By now I had married my girlfriend, and we had a young son. I was happy and living a normal life as a civilian.

The profession I had chosen was working in the public sector. It is a tough job with many lows, but these are outweighed by the high points.

For me moving to a new area was nothing new as this is part of the military lifestyle, but for my wife it was hard. It was the first time she had been so far away from family and friends, but we eventually settled down. She now has a good job that she enjoys and has made some good friends.

During this time, I did what we all do – struggle through life, rolling with the punches and just doing the best we can. Looking back in hindsight, I didn't realize what was starting to happen.

In my new community, I had no friends and no social life. All I did was go to work and then come home and flop in front of the TV. I was isolating myself from the world. Although I didn't know it, this was the beginning of my descent into the darkest of places.

Years of high stress and trauma were building, and I was completely unaware of the toll this was about to take. A tragic family bereavement involving a child was the trigger for my illness coming to the fore. I awoke one night with a start. My heart was pounding, my guts were churning, and I was soaked in sweat. I was so wet I thought I had wet myself. Worst of all, I was terrified, and I could not understand why.

I lay in the dark, scared and confused. I could not move; I wanted to get out of bed, but I couldn't. Although I was pouring with sweat, I could not get warm. I started to feel sick; I managed to get to the toilet and was violently ill from both ends. Not an easy thing to do by any means.

I did not know it at the time, but my body had gone into what's called "fight or flight." My brain was flooding my body with adrenaline and emptying my stomach and bowls ready to run or fight.

This went on for about five years. I had long periods of sick leave, night terrors, nightmares, insomnia, and forgetfulness, inability to concentrate – the list goes on.

Asking for help was not an option. Weakness is for the feeble. I saw myself as an alpha male, and I would get through this my way. What a load of crap. Eventually, I broke. I was diagnosed with delayed onset PTSD. A fantastic charity called Combat Stress took me into their care.

I spent six weeks in one of their recovery centers which are in effect psychiatric hospitals for veterans suffering from PTSD. While there I met some incredible people from all walks of life with all sorts of experiences. We all had one thing in common. We were losing our battle with PTSD. I soon learned that being exposed to trauma and coming through it was not a ceasefire. The battle was not over, far from it – it had only just begun. PTSD is relentless. It destroys relationships, careers, self-confidence and over time can destroy life. It is an injury I would not wish upon my worst enemies.

I cannot speak for those suffering from PTSD who haven't served in the armed forces, but I have realized that we veterans are different compared to people from other walks of life. We don't think like other people. We don't see the world like other people. When most people go for a walk in the countryside, they see rolling hills, lush woodlands, or flowing streams. We see firing points, contact points, and dead ground. We don't feel like other people because we don't feel. We are numb to feeling as the military has trained us to be this way.

You don't know me. I am next to you on the bus. I am the person standing behind you in the queue at the supermarket. I deliver your mail; I drive the taxi that takes you home after a good night out. I am the homeless guy in the doorway, pissed and asleep. I am the latest suicide you read about in your local paper. I am PTSD. It cannot be cured, but it can be understood. Like I have already said, I don't want sympathy. I see this injury as my cross to bear for the things I have done and those I have hurt. All I ask is please don`t judge us. After all, you may be happy in your world, but you never know what fate has in store.

If just one person reads this book and recognizes a bit of what they may be feeling and seeks help, then for me that will be job done, and I can stand down.

Soldier - No.5

Never the Same Again,
"Then Came the Call to Ireland,
As the Call Had Come Before,
Another Bloody Chapter,
In an Endless Civil War.

Harvey Andrews

Fighting a battle inside your head every single day is exhausting. Before I elaborate, let me go back and describe some of my background.

I was born into the Army, the son of a Warrant Officer. To say I had a disciplined upbringing would be an understatement. Comments such as "big boys and men don't cry" and "pull yourself together" were common. Joining the Army seemed like a natural progression after school. Our basic training, though tough for many, seemed second nature to me. I struggled to comprehend why people were 'homesick' at their age (most recruits were in their late teens and early twenties). Travelling the world with my parents and being sent to boarding schools had taught me how to cope with homesickness. I made friends easily and life was good.

My first posting was to the tropical climes of Wiltshire - deep joy! I soon settled, and life was a conveyor belt of long shifts and parties aplenty. I had money in my pocket, friends, a great life   I was living the dream.
Then in 1985 I received a posting order to Northern Ireland. Life as I knew it was about to change. I had very little knowledge about exactly what was going on in Ulster - I'd never been particularly interested in

politics or the history of Northern Ireland. Of course, I was aware there was civil unrest, murders, shootings, bombings and riots and that this had been going on since 1969. Notwithstanding that, the reality of the situation became apparent very quickly.

My very first patrol of West Belfast introduced me to the intense feelings of hatred towards the British Army. It was like nothing I had ever experienced before, and no amount of training could have prepared me. The look of mistrust, disgust and downright hatred in the eyes of the residents, young and old alike, was clearly apparent. Seeing some of the women spitting in our direction left quite an impression on my young mind. We shrugged it off though, and wanting to maintain normal life, we joked around on a regular basis. Most service personnel did tours of NI for 3-6 months. In my case, like many others, I was there for two and a half years.

In all that time, my brain became conditioned into a certain way of thinking. I suspected everyone not in the Forces, and if there wasn't outright mistrust, there was an element of suspicion towards everyone I meet. I checked my vehicle for Improvised Explosive Devices (IED) daily - vigilance was paramount. My stories and experiences from that time are numerous. Many are comical, but several are hauntingly frightening and two will be forever etched in my brain. I see no need to go into detail (I have done that to the psychiatrists, therapists, and counsellors). Suffice it to say that these experiences involved extreme violence and I feel lucky to be here writing now.

I say lucky, although there have been occasions over the years where I didn't feel so lucky and thought about taking my own life. The effect those experiences and incidents had on me are now only too apparent. In hindsight, it is apparent that my character started to change immediately following these incidents. For a while I had the most awful nightmares. I was snappy with people, behaved irrationally, and my mistrust of others even began to extend to friends and colleagues.

As time passed though, I buried those thoughts and life settled for me. Although I wasn't consciously aware of the change, my drinking had increased tenfold. Posted to Germany, I drank heavily to escape memories and argued constantly with my wife. I threw myself into work and the gym - when I wasn't doing that I was drinking in the Mess with the lads. I was busy enough, but my marriage that suffered. I just didn't want to be around someone who kept asking questions about how I was doing. Without a doubt, I was selfish. I suffered a serious injury in 1988 and following several operations, I was casualty evacuated back to the UK.

I underwent several more major operations in The Queen Elizabeth Military Hospital, Woolwich and with so much time to just lie in bed and think, the inevitable happened. The nightmares started up again, accompanied this time by flashbacks in the daytime. Repeatedly I relived the most intense and dangerous moments from Northern Ireland as though I was still there.

On Christmas Eve 1989, the Army Chaplain came to the Hospital ward to visit the six or seven of us who remained there for Christmas. He asked if any of us would like to attend Midnight Mass that night. Seeing this as an opportunity to unburden myself and get some help, I asked if I could be pushed down to the Chapel and whether I could speak privately with the Chaplain following the service. All was arranged. I can't really remember details about the service, but it was well attended by nurses, patients from other wards and staff. When the service ended people filtered out slowly, some nodding their heads at me as I lay in my bed at the back.

The Chaplain approached when the place was empty. He sat on my bed and said: "What's troubling you, Sergeant?"

All I could do was breakdown completely and sob uncontrollably. He took my hand and gripping it tightly said: "It's alright son. I've had bigger and harder men than you do this before."

I don't know how long I was there, but I do recall waking up back on the ward on Christmas morning. What happened a few days later stunned me? I was visited by a doctor (a captain, if I recall) and he was accompanied by several other doctors.

He entered the ward and in a loud voice said: "Right, Sergeant, what's all this about you blubbing on the Padre's shoulder?"

I was mortified and fully aware that several people (patients and staff) were looking at me. From that point onwards, it was a spiral downwards for me. I decided to bury all mention of my past experiences. Although apparently, I'd developed a knack for pissing off officers, which followed me for the remainder of my military career. I just didn't care about how other people felt. If I thought something, I'd say it. As for trusting anyone with knowledge or information about me – forget it!

I left the Army in 1994 but the past has a habit of catching up with you (or never really leaving you, despite what people believe). I'd remarried but the transition to civilian life had not run smoothly. Everything was felt alien – the humor (or lack of it), work ethics and more. I struggled to find true camaraderie. I missed the military way of life enormously. My drinking continued in abundance. Any time there were external stressors, my mind went into overdrive and the only crutch I had was alcohol.

Eventually I joined Her Majesty's Prison Service (HMPS), a disciplined, hierarchical organisations - sound familiar? Here I found the camaraderie I had missed, as many of the other 'Screws' were ex-Forces as well. There was plenty to keep me busy too. Prison is an active environment and despite now being in my 40s, my mind still functioned as though I was in my 20s. My military training came to the fore, helping me to settle into my new career. However, with this sort of physical job, there also came drawbacks. Many convicts doing their time have mental health issues too. Acting as part of a team to restrain these guys or dealing with the aftermath of an attempted (or successful suicide) began to take its toll.

A major trigger in a complete breakdown I suffered was the suicide of a close friend of mine. He was also a Prison Officer, but his death stunned many of us and I was catapulted into deep depression. Memories from my past in Northern Ireland resurfaced and I suffered many of the now quite well-known symptoms of PTSD - flashbacks, nightmares, hypervigilance. From the outside, it's easy to imagine that after a certain amount of time, memories fade and trauma gets relegated to the past. Sadly, with PTSD nothing fades. Our bodies and brains will not let us forget because of surging chemicals that reinforce every memory.

We cannot just walk away from the past. As we are operating on a kind of autopilot we are not always in control. PTSD is an exaggerated state of survival mode and we experience emotions that frighten and overwhelm even us. We simply cannot stop the anger, tears and other destructive and disruptive behaviors that are so difficult for others to understand. The thing about anxiety and depression is that they are co-morbid diagnoses with PTSD.

I recall taking one of my sons to play rugby. We were driving down the A1 (M) to St Neots but after several minutes I noticed a green MG enter the traffic from a slip road and pull in behind me. Immediately I felt my pulse quicken and my breathing became shallower and more rapid. My lad was aged about 12 at the time and the mood in the car had been one of happiness and we'd been laughing and joking until this point. I saw that there were two males in the car, but it was the way it had maneuver into the traffic behind me that had caused my reaction. I decided to slow down and took my foot off the accelerator. The MG slowed down. I accelerated and tried to pull away, the MG did the same and by now, my lad had noticed that something wasn't quite right.

"Dad, what's the matter?"

"Nothing son." I replied although by my very actions he became scared.

I told him that we were going to take a little diversion and with that, I overtook the car in front of me and then cut back across two lanes and took the slip road off the motorway. I recall my feelings and emotions at the time. I was ready take on anybody for bringing my kids into danger and there was going to be major trouble, bastards!! Although my man oeuvre had been quick, the MG managed to follow us down the slip road. I accelerated even more and didn't stop at the end of the slip road. I took a couple of turns downside roads and then came to an abrupt stop. I watched in the rear-view mirror as the MG went driving past the end of the road, clearly looking for us. My son was shaken and tearful, but I reassured him that everything was going to be fine and we made our way to the rugby club. As we pulled into the car park, I saw the green MG immediately and was approached by a man who turned out to be one of the dads taking his son to play in the same game. He'd recognise my car and as he was unfamiliar with where St Neots rugby club was, he thought he follow me.

What had I done? I'd just terrified my 12-year-old through some irrational thoughts I'd had that IRA were coming after me. My doctor diagnosed me with the clinical depression, and I was off work for five months living on medication and alcohol. My wife and I separated, and I found myself living in a bedsit with nothing but time on my hands. It was a recipe for disaster. I was sent to see a counsellor and over a 5-month period, she saw me weekly. There wasn't any other medical intervention and although I had some support from friends, the Prison Service informed me that unless I returned to work, I would only receive half salary at the 6-month point.

Ultimately, I buried my feelings. It took me several attempts to return to work, but things settled once more and I 'just got on with it'. Through more injuries (sustained at work) over the ensuing years, I was medically retired from work in 2015. Once again with so much time on my hands following yet more surgery and my spinal condition worsening, chronic pain led me to 'that dark place'.

It was in 2014 that I first heard of the organisation Combat Stress. Over the years, I've recognised that I have a major problem and I have asked for help. However, the Army in those days didn't want to know. If you weren't A1 fit, you were malingering or a problem. Of course, because of our training and backgrounds, it may be that we didn't help ourselves by keeping everything bottled up either. Additionally, many general practitioners and health professionals do not have the necessary understanding of PTSD and need further education.

Last year in June 2015 after drinking half a bottle of vodka, I took the plunge and called Combat Stress. The help I have received since then has been phenomenal. After an initial visit and assessment by an outreach CPN, I attended a 2-week stabilisation program. The next year I participated in a 6-week Residential Intensive Treatment Program at Tyrwhitt House run by Combat Stress. It's extremely difficult revisiting the past. However, it was the job of the staff at Combat Stress to stir up those memories I spent so long trying to bury – it has been an uncomfortable journey.

Simply visiting shops, leaving my home, being invited to social events and even answering the telephone has on many occasions been impossible. Likewise, with social gatherings and invitations - I have cancelled so many of those that people no longer ask me. I have great difficulty in seeing the world as I experienced it before my traumas. Now I see every moment as dangerous, unpredictable and threatening.

Why is helping ex service personnel predominantly left to charities? Does our government not care about the sacrifices we have made during our service?

A soldier with PTSD fell in a hole and despite trying for a long time, he couldn't get out. A senior NCO walked by and the soldier with PTSD called out for help. The SNCO yelled at him, told him to suck it up, dig deep and drive on, then he threw him a shovel. The soldier tried but he couldn't just suck it up and drive on, so he used the shovel, but the hole got deeper. A senior Officer walked by and the soldier called out for help. "Use the tools your SNCO gave you," said the Officer and he threw him a bucket to try and help. The soldier thought,"...but I AM using the tools my SNCO gave me, it's not working!!" He then tried to use the bucket but all it was good for was filling with earth. A well-known psychiatrist walked by and the soldier cried: "Help!! I can't get out." The psychiatrist threw down some drugs and said: "Take these; they'll relieve the anxiety and the pain." The soldier said thanks but when the pills ran out, he was STILL in the hole. A psychologist was next to pass by and he heard the soldier's cries for help. He stopped and asked: "How did you get in there? Were you born there? Did your parents put you in there? Tell me all about yourself; it will alleviate your sense of loneliness and hopelessness." So, the soldier talked with him but after an hour, the psychologist said he had to leave although he'd be back next week. The soldier thanked him, but he was STILL in the hole!! A priest had heard about the soldier, so he came to see him. He talked and gave him a Bible and said: "I'll say a prayer for you." He got down on his knees next to the hole and they prayed together. Then he too, had to leave. The soldier with PTSD was very grateful and thanked the priest and then he read the Bible. When he finished reading, he realised that he was STILL stuck in the hole. After a while, a recovering soldier with PTSD happened to be passing by. The soldier in the hole cried out: "Hey, help me. I'm stuck in this hole!!" Right away, the recovering soldier with PTSD jumped down into the hole with him. The soldier said: "What are you doing? Now we're both stuck down here!" But the recovering soldier with PTSD put his arm around his shoulder and said: "Calm down, it's okay. I've been down here before. I know how to get out.!" ¬ Author unknown

Soldier - No.6

You cannot patch a wounded
soul with a Band-Aid.
The Fresh Quotes

For security reasons, I've changed some of the dates, times and names in the following account.

I joined the army as a Junior Leader at the end of 1985. I joined my battalion in Germany at the end of 1986. I completed a couple of military courses and took part in overseas exercises in UK and Canada. My military career was excellent apart from an event in which a very close friend was killed by a German taxi driver. Like most squaddies, my time in Germany consisted of barrack life or drinking plenty of beer on the weekends.

In 1988, my battalion was sent to Northern Ireland, OP BANNER, for a two-year posting. This is where things went badly wrong for me. Northern Ireland currently was at the height of the Troubles.

When we landed in Northern Ireland, my company went straight on the ground to the borders of East Tyrone (Bandit Country). We manned checkpoints and spent a huge amount of time patrolling. On one of my first patrols, we'd been out for a couple of days when we came across an old abandoned farm. The farm was overgrown and tumbling down. It was winter and freezing cold. That night the whole patrol slept in an old barn. Just as it was getting dark, I was poking around the yard when I stumbled across an old railway guard's carriage behind a mound of soil and weeds in the far corner of the yard. It seemed odd, but I guessed that being an old farm anything would look odd to me. The first half of the carriage was full of bottles of Position (Irish Distilled Beverage, 40% - 90% abv), and a couple of bottles managed to end up coming with us. The other half of the carriage was open and had a rust hole in the wriggly tin roof. The carriage was full of nettles, but in the middle of the floorboards there was a hole. The nettles were dead and dried around the hole. I took a wee in the hole, and I noticed six corroded metallic cylinders stacked up where the boards had rotted away. I pee'd on them and then went on, not thinking much more about the cylinders. The next morning, we patrolled out of the farm. Three or four days later back at the RUC station, we debriefed, and that was that.

Due to my skillset, I was often called to head out on patrol with other units. Thanks to courses I'd done previously I was mainly attached to the signal's guys. A good friend from another company was also doing the same type of work as me. I loved every minute of what I was doing, but I now know that I most like shouldn't have been doing it and was well out of my depth on several occasions.

About a year and a half into the posting, I was on the way out of a Royal Ulster Constabulary station with three other guys to check monitoring devices on illegal border crossing points. I only ever knew one bloke's name, Brian. I'd been out with them 7 or 8 times on the ground, so we sort of knew how each person operated in the field.

We were on the way out to the guard room when one of the guys said: "Bugger, I've left --------- (a classified piece of electrical equipment) in my room."

His room was down the end of a long corridor. I said: "No worries, I'll go and get it."

I never saw those blokes again. As I jogged back to the guardroom, I heard a huge BOOOOOM. The blast blew me backward down the corridor. I hit my back on a drink vending machine. It was the third mortar attack that week. The smells and sights of that moment are burnt into my mind, and they flash before my eyes every second of every day.

I was cast vac to a military wing in a hospital in Northern Ireland, then on to Queen Elizabeth Military Hospital in Woolwich, London. I thought my Army days were over for sure. I was in Woolwich for approximately three weeks. I didn't know what to expect or what was going to happen.

One day towards the end of my stay in Woolwich, three gentlemen came walking down the corridor towards my bed space. Two of them were in uniform and the other one in a suit. I was asked: "Are you L/Cpl?"

I looked at them in confusion and said: "Yes."

Was I going to be medically discharged or something?

The bloke in the suit then turned, looked at me and said: "We need to ask you about something you found on the farm back in while on patrol."

I instantly knew what they were going on about. It transpired that some bloke somewhere was burning old patrol reports. As he was turning page after page (it's a dull job, I've done it myself), he noticed my Platoon Commander's last entry: "Pte located six unusual metal objects in the farmyard. "

I didn't get to see the report myself, but the bloke burning the reports recognized it as something they had been looking for. I have never written a patrol report, but as far as I was aware all grid references and coordinates had already been destroyed.

As I was free, they offered me the opportunity to go back out with another regiment. Like a dick, I jumped at the chance. A couple of weeks later I was attached to a subunit in Bulford. We trained together for three weeks, then got airlifted back to Northern Ireland. I'm not sure where exactly we were; it was a small compound but bloody busy RUC station. We stayed there overnight sorting out equipment. Late afternoon the following day we were picked up in two transit vans which drove for a couple of hours. The two vans stopped at a small dilapidated part-time RUC station. I didn't know where we were or who opened the gate. The five of us ran into the compound and slammed the door behind us, and the vans sped off into the night.

The villagers seemed to have been throwing petrol bombs at the RUC Station building for months. We stayed the night and most of the following day. We slept and ate egg banjos from what was left in the fridge. The village looked quaint, with no streetlights. The nearest house was along a ridge about 400 yards from our location. As night fell, we left through the back gate into a sort of maze of tin sheets and barbed wire. It stank of fuel and smoke, and the ground was covered in broken glass.

I stepped out of a hole in the sheeting and followed the other four guys. I looked back at the silhouette of the RUC station; it was black and angry looking. At that time, I had no idea that the bed I had slept in for the past few nights would be the last bed I'd sleep in for nearly eight months. Our job was to search every single grid square in the entire area of East Tyrone until I found the farm again. We had food and water dropped off by helicopters; this would become a normal routine. The five of us had secure radio nets to avoid being caught by the IRA.

We had a couple of very near misses. On one occasion PIRA was playing football for 10 minutes or what felt like a lifetime about 20 yards from my lay-up position. That was scary as hell. We were all made ready in case of a shootout or better known as a hit and run.

Most of the time we saw or came across nothing. Approximately nine weeks after the football incident, it was late spring. We walked into a surreal scene with the oddest plants I saw in my life. They were alien and huge, at least 12 feet high and with hollow stems, a bit like rhubarb. We patrolled in through a gap in the leaves. Straight away I recognized the roof of the barn where my patrol had slept nearly two years ago. This was the place without any doubt. I signaled "enemy" because to be honest I felt excited about finding the place. Our patrol got down into all-round defense, and one of the guys went to check the area out.

From this point onwards it all turned to shit for me. One of the members of the patrol got on the radio. I didn't hear the message that was sent over the net but approximately 20 minutes later two RAF Wessex helicopters appeared. They landed in the field running parallel to the corner of the farmyard along to the barn where we slept all two years ago. Suddenly loads of blokes jumped out of these two helicopters. Half of the personnel were in full hazmat coveralls and oxygen cylinders. What the fuck had I found two years ago? Some of the guys in plainclothes talked to three of the four guys from our patrol again. Approximately 20 minutes later three or four Landrovers and a flatbed lorry came bombing up the well-overgrown track. As the first Landrover came into the farmyard, it ran over those strange plants. They made a loud hollow popping sound; I never heard a noise like it since.

I don't know what regiment jumped out of these Landrovers but they started pulling big sheets of Harris fencing off the flatbed under direction of the guys in hazmat kit. While this was going on, I asked one of the four guys what was happening. He spoke to an officer in one of the Landovers who pointed at one of the

Wessex helicopters. There must have been about 40+ men on the ground by this point.

I was waiting for the pat on the back and was told: "Well done, lad, you did well. Get on the Wessex, and off you go!"

The terminology was a bit more colorful than that, but you get the idea. I shook hands with the guys and did what I was told.

The Wessex took me to RAF Aldergrove. I went to the guardroom as directed. It must have been about 1600hrs by this time. I handed my GPMG and 9mm Browning in as directed. They informed me they didn't want my ammo which was a bit odd, but I just got onto the waiting Hercules with about 30 other soldiers and flew to RAF Lyneham. I was picked up off the Hercules by Landover and dropped off at the guardroom with the others from the patrol.

The duty sergeant said: "Ah L/Cpl, I understand you have ammunition for me?"

I handed over all my ammo. He gave me a rail warrant and said: "Cheers, then."

I walked out towards the gate and asked the bloke on stag: "Now what?" He just laughed.

So, I walked for a couple of hours, and a bloke pulled up and offered me a lift to Paddington station. I got my ticket from the ticket office in exchange for my rail warrant and got on my way home.

Unfortunately, the train wasn't stopping at my town and went to the city, which was about 12 miles by road from my town and about 8 miles over the hills. I decided for the hills and headed that way. It was a crisp, clear moonlit night. I had bought a house a couple of years earlier and was renting out a room out to an ex-Royal Marine. He was visiting his girlfriend in Plymouth, so the house was empty when I arrived home. It was around 0420hrs when I got to my front door. I dug up the spare key and managed to get in.

I stood for a while in dead silence of my house. I don't know how long I stood there. I felt numb, shell-shocked. I took my Bergen rucksack off and dropped it to the floor in the hallway. I dumped my webbing on top of it. I got out of the stinking clothes I'd been wearing for seven months. I hadn't washed or shaved in all that time, nor had I seen a bed. Less than 12 hours before I'd been patrolling in a very hostile environment. Now I was alone, overwhelmed by the feeling of *what the fuck do I do now?*

I had a little cry. Then I just tried to deal with my feelings and get on with my life. Several months later I got a letter from the barracks in Bulford saying that I had to collect my MFO box and hand in all issued kit. My career in the army had ended.

I was diagnosed with chronic PTSD in mid-2013. The bloke who came out to assess me said in his parting breath: "Your main problem is that you are still 'stood too!' "

The odd thing is, I'd never thought of it before. I muttered under my breath as he left: "No shit!"

I've had a couple of residential stays at Combat Stress in Leatherhead in Surrey in 2015 and 2016. I've only told a handful of people this stuff and everyone has gone "WHAT?" and "Jesus WTF" but then I met a gentleman at Combat Stress who was ex Royal Navy and worked on nuclear class submarines during the Cold War. He was a very nice chap, and I was in a talkative mood that afternoon. I told him about the find and he said: "I'll stop you there, I know what you found."

My experiences over the past 20 years have resulted in hypervigilance, depression, isolation, inability to switch off or relax, fear, inability to sleep due to (I hate this word) flashbacks, survival guilt and a feeling of worthlessness about myself and my lack of trust in others.

I feel much messed up and let down. I am always on edge. I am tired, worn out. I just want it to stop and go away. Because of PTSD I've lost my family, my home, my job and my self-worth and self-respect. Someone made a glib remark a while ago: "Oh, but I bet you would not do it again, would you?"

Conclusion

During the writing of this book I came up against many obstacles blocking my attempts to research specific information regarding combat stress and PTSD. It seems that governments don't want their citizens to know that many soldiers return home from war suffering mental health injuries.

While suffering from insomnia (another symptom of PTSD) and researching this book I came across a film called *Let There Be Light* (1946). To my surprise, I discovered this film was banned in the USA until 1981. When I watched the film, I could see why it had been banned. The film vividly told the truth about wounded soldiers suffering from mental health injures upon their return home from war. As stated in the movie, 20% of American service personnel returning home from World War Two suffered from mental health conditions.

If this film had been widely released in 1946, it would have shocked the nation, and Americans would have demanded further information and treatment for the soldiers and veterans. The film might have made its way it way to the UK and could have encouraged people there to learn more about shell shock or mental health. But banning this movie continued the stigma around mental health and allowed for governments to deny the existence of combat stress until 40 years later. We may never receive an answer as to why powerful governments like the USA and UK wanted to deny the existence of mental health injuries in soldiers and thus hinder their treatment. However, it is time for change to happen.

There are no clear answers as to why only some people suffer from PTSD, but its existence cannot be denied. Some people will be open to diagnosis and treatment and be willing to support others. Some people continue to simply say there no such thing as PTSD. If there was a cure for PTSD, then the many people suffering from it would leap at the chance – I know I would. All we ask is to be treated like normal people with a heart, feelings and the need to be heard and understood.

Printed in Great Britain
by Amazon

35527887R00083